Homemade Cleaners

45 DIY Cleaners Based on Essential Oil

TABLE OF CONTENTS

Introduction 5

Chapter 1. Cleaning Products Are Effecting Our Health 6

Chapter 2. Homemade Non-Toxic Cleaning Products 8
   1. *Homemade Laundry Detergent (powder)*..8
   2. *Homemade Fabric Softener (for dryer)* 9
   3. *Fabric Softener (washing machine)* 10
   4. *Shower Spray* 11
   5. *Homemade "Comet"* 12
   6. *Toilet Bowl Cleaner* 13
   7. *Glass & Mirror Cleaner* 14
   8. *Homemade Carpet Freshener*... 15
   9. *Homemade Room Spray* 16
   10. *All Purpose Cleaner #1* 17
   11. *All Purpose Cleaner #2*... 18

Chapter 2. All Natural Bath & Beauty Products... 19
   12. *Coconut Salt Scrub*.. 21
   13. *Whipped Coconut Oil Lotion*...22
   14. *Body Wash* 23
   15. *Shaving Cream #1*...24
   16. *Shaving Cream #2* 25
   17. *Energizing Body Spray*..26
   18. *Foaming Hand Soap*..27
   19. *Vanilla & Lavender Detoxing Bath Salts* 28
   20. *Foaming Face Wash*...29
   21. *Bubble Bath* 30

Chapter 3. Aromatherapy Essential Oil Blends.. 31
   22. *Fresh and Clean Essential Oil Diffuser Recipe*...............................34

23. *Seasonal Allergies Essential Oil Diffuser Recipe* 35

24. *Flower Garden Essential Oil Diffuser Recipe* 36

25. *Morning Boost Essential Oil Diffuser Recipe* 37

26. *Cold and Flu Season Essential Oil Diffuser Recipe* 38

27. *Focus and Alertness Essential Oil Diffuser Recipe* 39

28. *Odor Eliminator Essential Oil Diffuser Recipe* 40

Chapter 4. DIY Budget Friendly Cleaning Products 41

29. *Vinyl & Linoleum* 41

30. *Dusting Spray* 42

31. *Wood Polish* 43

32. *Simple Dusting Spray* 44

Chapter 5. Teeth Cleaners & More! 45

33. *Squeezable Toothpaste for Clean Teeth* 45

34. *Teeth Whitening Scrub* 46

35. *Detox Bath Recipe* 47

36. *Detox Hair Mask* 48

37. *Powerful Essential Oil Blend for Toenail Fungus* 49

38. *Foot Soak* 50

39. *Healing Blend for Acne Scars* 51

40. *Pumpkin Spice Scrub Cubes* 52

41. *Exfoliating Lip Scrub* 53

42. *Tea Tree Dandruff Shampoo* 54

43. *Facial Mist for Radiant Skin* 55

44. *Foaming Citrus Body Wash* 56

45. *Skin Clearing Facial Mask* 57

Conclusion 58

FREE Bonus Reminder 59

Introduction

I would first like to thank and congratulate you on downloading *"Essential Oil Cleaners: Homemade Essential Oil Based Cleaning Products for Household and Personal Use."* You are going to love making your own homemade cleaning products, especially when you see the money this is going to save you and that they are environmentally friendly. Making your own homemade cleaning products is a great example to set for your children, showing them that making your own homemade products is better for you and the environment. This can teach your children to have respect for their surroundings by using products that are environmentally friendly.

What is great about making your own cleaning products is that you can get creative and add in your favorite essential oils to make it a special personal blend of your own. Use your imagination to create some fun essential oil based cleaning products. You can use the recipes in this book, but you can also add to them to make a recipe your own. Adding a special ingredient to a recipe to give it that extra boost that you are looking for.

Chapter 1. Cleaning Products Are Effecting Our Health

The last thing that any of us wants to believe is that the cleaning products that we have been using for many years to help us to keep our home environment clean could be causing us more harm than good. The serious harm that cleaning products could be causing is only recently being researched in an in-depth level. Our generation has certainly seen an increase in infertility, asthma, cancer and thyroid disease. Researchers are beginning to connect the dots regarding these ailments and our enormous exposure to harmful chemicals. We are exposed to toxic metals, pesticides, environmental pollution, toxic plastics, artificial food, just to name a few. The elevated level of harmful chemicals being used daily is the reason that researching the effect on the human body has been very challenging to conduct.

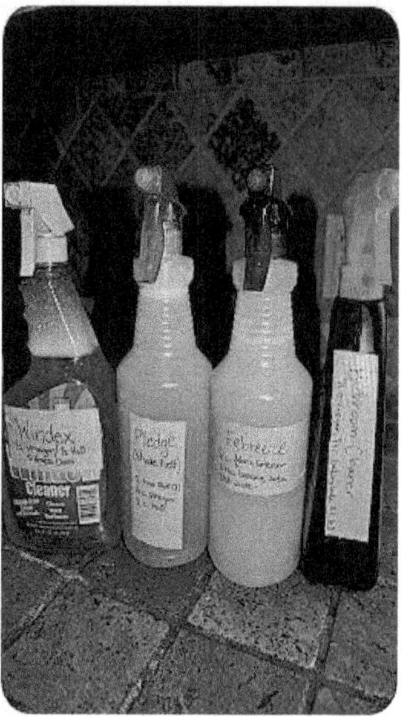

Many mainstream cleaning products have been identified as being major culprits in affecting our health. Slowly over time we are exposed to these harmful chemicals. Harmful chemicals can be found in many of today's cleaning products on the market. They can basically be divided into three categories, namely carcinogens, neurotoxins, and endocrine disruptors.

1. **Carcinogens** are dangerous cancer causing substances, that directly affect our bodies at a cellular level.

2. **Neurotoxins** are very destructive and can cause damage to our nerve tissue, which can potentially have negative effects on our concentration, memory, and sleeping patterns.

3. **Endocrine Disruptors** cause disruption with our hormone systems, this in turn can cause our bodies to react in an erratic manner to these mixed signals.

You might even have a feeling or sense of betrayal by those cleaning products that you have used for many years to clean your home environment. Most us have been lulled into believing that the cleaning products sold on the mainstream market are all safe to use. We believe that if they were not that the authorities would certainly not allow them to be sold on the open market. We don't want to think that the authorities would knowingly allow companies to produce products that could be responsible for causing serious diseases. The sad truth is that many companies are driven by the greed of profit. The authorities cannot do anything unless they have solid proof that a specific substance is a health risk.

Not only are many of the cleaning products on the market very harmful to our health, but they are also very detrimental to the environment as well. Most aerosol spray cans contain CFC's that cause harm to the ozone layer and they contribute to the greenhouse effect. Our future is leading us towards a global water crisis, adding to this awful crisis will be toxic substances from cleaning products finding their way into our sensitive water systems, causing great harm to our natural resources on a large scale long after you wash them down your sink.

To help to provide a healthier environment you must take action against the mainstream cleaning products. Acting against harmful cleaning products will help to ensure the long-term wellbeing of yourself and loved ones.

Good News:

The good news is that it is not difficult to go green. You will certainly enjoy the health benefits and peace of mind, that you will get from using natural cleaning products that are also very cost effective. You will be able to customize your own homemade products to suit your personal needs. This book is "green-based," containing green recipes, 100% safe to use around your kids and pets, they have eco friendly ingredients that will cause you no harm or the environment.

Chapter 2. Homemade Non-Toxic Cleaning Products

1. Homemade Laundry Detergent (powder)

Ingredients:

- 1 cup baking soda

- 1 cup washing soda

- 1 bar of castile soap or natural soap of your choice

- 1 cup of borax

- ½ cup of all natural laundry whitener

- 15 drops of lavender, lemon or lime essential oil

- Sealable container

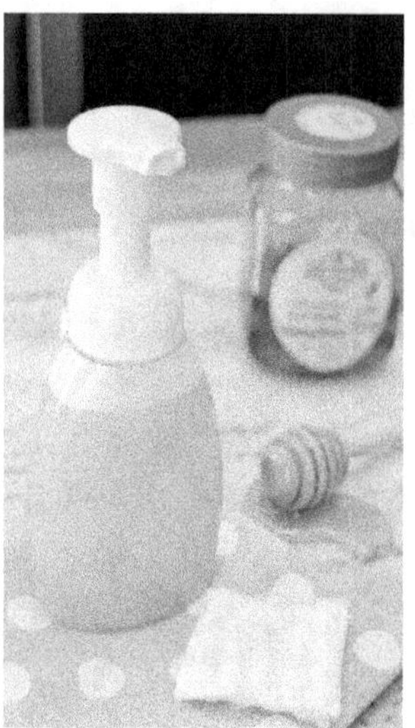

Directions:

Run the bar of soap through your food processor grater attachment. Add other ingredients, except for the essential oils. Mix until soap and powders are well blended. Add in your essential oils and blend for another 30 seconds. Transfer the mixture to sealable container and use 1-2 tablespoons per load.

2. Homemade Fabric Softener (for dryer)
Ingredients:

- 5 cut up J-clothes or sponges or old tea towels or t-shirts
- 30 drops of your favorite essential oil
- 2 cups of vinegar
- Sealable container

Directions:

Place the rags into your container and add vinegar and essential oils. Wring out one rag at a time and add to your load in the dryer. When your clothes are dried place the rag back into the container.

3. Fabric Softener (washing machine)
Ingredients:

- Vinegar- fill container with vinegar
- 20 drops of your favorite essential oil
- Small pourable container

Directions:

Fill the pourable container with vinegar and add in the essential oils. Stir until well blended. Add this mixture to your fabric softener dispenser of your washing machine.

4. *Shower Spray*

Ingredients:

- 1 cup of castile soap
- 1 cup of vinegar
- 1 cup of water
- 15 drops of essential oil

Directions:

Mix all your ingredients in a spray bottle. After you have finished scrubbing your shower with some homemade "comet" (comet recipe next), use this spray after each shower.

5. Homemade "Comet"

Ingredients:

- ½ cup of Borax
- 2 cups baking soda
- 10 drops of tea tree essential oil
- 10 drops of lemon essential oil

Directions:

Mix ingredients in a bowl and pour into an empty parmesan cheese container for storage.

6. *Toilet Bowl Cleaner*

Ingredients:

- ¼ cup vinegar
- 1 cup hot water
- 10 drops of lavender essential oil
- ¼ cup of hydrogen peroxide
- ½ cup of baking soda
- ¼ cup castile soap

Directions:

Mix the castile soap and baking soda together. Add in the essential oils and peroxide. Slowly add in hot water. Stir in vinegar, until foaming stops. Pour mix into a squeeze top bottle. Squeeze the mix around the inside rim of toilet and let sit for 10 minutes before you scrub the toilet with toilet brush.

7. Glass & Mirror Cleaner

Ingredients:

- 15 drops of lemon essential oil
- 1 tablespoon of cornstarch (will reduce the streaks)
- ¼ cup of rubbing alcohol
- ¼ cup vinegar

Directions:

Mix all your ingredients into a spray bottle. Shake well before each use.

8. Homemade Carpet Freshener

Ingredients:

- 2 cups of baking soda

- 20 drops of orange essential oil

- Shakeable sealable container (I find empty parmesan cheese shaker works well)

Directions:

Mix your essential oils and baking soda in container. Sprinkle on carpet or other fabrics, allow it to sit for about 20 minutes then vacuum.

9. Homemade Room Spray

Ingredients:

- 15 drops of lavender essential oil
- 2 cups of distilled water
- 1 tablespoon of baking soda
- Empty spray bottle

Directions:

Add your ingredients into empty sprat bottle, and shake before each use.

10. All Purpose Cleaner #1

Ingredients:

- 1 teaspoon of borax
- ¼ cup of vinegar
- 2 tablespoons of Castile soap
- 15 drops of tea tree or lemon essential oil
- Warm water

Directions:

Pour the borax and vinegar into the spray bottle. Swirl until dissolved. Fill bottle up with warm water and shake. Add in the essential oils and Castile soap and shake. Shake before each use.

11. All Purpose Cleaner #2

Ingredients:

- Vinegar

- 20 drops of lemon or tea tree essential oil

- Spray bottle

Directions:

Fill the spray bottle with vinegar and essential oils. Use this mixture to clean kitchen, bathroom and any surfaces.

Chapter 2. All Natural Bath & Beauty Products

Cleaning products that we use on our skin have a direct effect on our health. Cleaning products such as shampoos, conditioners, creams and cleansers have ingredients in them that penetrate our skin. The dermis is penetrated by about 60% of chemicals

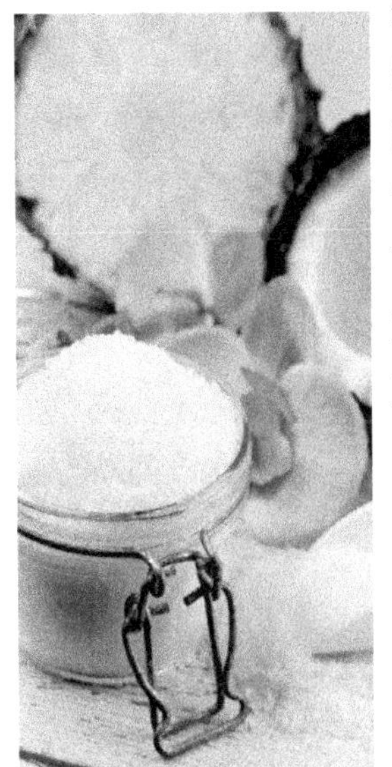

found in major body cleaning products. These are absorbed into the lower layers of our skin, and even getting into our bloodstream. We often use the ability for our skin to absorb things to help deliver medications quickly through the skin. You can use this great ability of your skin to absorb healthy products rather than poisoning it with chemical-filled products.

Making your own natural skin care products is far superior to using personal care products that are on the market. Many products have been scientifically linked to harmful diseases and adverse effects on the human body.

Most product labels are very difficult to read, and few people understand what many of the ingredients are anyway. By using natural products, you will eliminate the dangers. Below are a few chemicals that are often found in personal products on the market today.

Heavy Metals

There has been imported skin lightening and anti-aging creams that have been found to contain toxic levels of mercury and other heavy metals. Several brands were discovered by the FDA investigations of these products. Mercury, can appear under different names such as "mercurous chloride" or "calomel." Aluminum is used in most personal care products, but especially it is found in deodorants. This is cause for great concern for women as aluminum has an estrogen-like effect that can cause disruption with the endocrine system and the underarm is close to the breasts.

Artificial Colors

The ingredients used in many personal care products to make them look more appealing can also be harmful to your health. Dyes such as D&C Red 27 and FD&C blue 1 are petroleum-based colours that have been suspected to cause cancer in humans. They have been banned in the European Union, but still are widely used in North America.

Triclosan

This is a product that has been in the news lately, it is the chemical used in many antibacterial soaps. Research has shown that it may cause bacteria to become antibiotic resistant and it can also disrupt thyroid and reproductive hormones.

Sodium lauryl sulfate (SLS) & Sodium laureth sulfate (SLES)

These are often used in foaming products such as body wash, acne treatment, shampoos, and face washes. Over 90 percent of personal care and cleaning products have these chemicals in them. When they are combined with other chemicals they can form a carcinogen.

Using essential oils can provide you with a safe non-toxic alternative. Essential oils come from plants, not petroleum, and they are effective because they permeate our tissues and are compatible with our cell structure. Products for beauty, bath, skincare, and household cleaning should be made with pure essential oils to eliminate the synthetic preservations, artificial fragrances, toxins, and artificial colours.

Essential oils will offer a safe and effective alternative to chemical products. Natural skincare is both safer and healthier for your skin.

12. Coconut Salt Scrub

Ingredients:

- 1 cup of coconut oil
- 2 teaspoons of Vitamin E oil
- ½ cup of Epsom salt
- 4 drops of lavender essential oil

Directions:

In a bowl mix the coconut oil and salt. Add in the essential oils and mix well. Store in a glass or plastic container and use in your bath or shower as an exfoliator.

13. Whipped Coconut Oil Lotion

Ingredients:

- 1 cup of coconut oil
- 10 drops of favorite essential oil
- 1 teaspoon of Vitamin E oil

Directions:

Add all the ingredients into a glass bowl and mix well. Using a hand mixer whip. Keep in a sealable glass container and store it in a cool place.

14. Body Wash
Ingredients:

- 15 drops of your favorite essential oil
- 1 teaspoon vegetable glycerine
- 1 cup water
- ¼ cup of Castile soap (you can use scented or unscented)

Directions:

Mix ingredients in a mixing bowl, then pour them into a squeeze bottle and use with a loofah puff.

15. Shaving Cream #1
Ingredients:

- 1 teaspoon of Vitamin E oil
- ¾ cup of Aloe Vera Gel
- ¼ cup of coconut oil
- 15 drops of your favorite essential oil

Directions:

Melt your ingredients in a double broiler, except for aloe, and essential oils. Remove from heat and add in the aloe, and essential oils and stir. Add mixture to plastic pump or squeeze bottle.

16. Shaving Cream #2

Ingredients:

- ¼ cup of unscented Castile soap
- ¼ cup honey
- ½ cup of olive, almond or grapeseed oil
- 15 drops of your favorite essential oil

Directions:

Combine ingredients in a bowl and whisk until emulsified. Transfer mixture into pump or squeeze bottle.

17. Energizing Body Spray

Ingredients:

- 5 drops of lavender essential oil
- 15 drops of grapefruit essential oil
- 1 tablespoon of witch hazel
- 5 ounces of distilled water

Directions:

Mix all the ingredients in a bowl and then add into a spray bottle. Shake well before each use.

18. Foaming Hand Soap

Ingredients:

- Water
- Unscented Castile soap
- 15 drops of your favorite essential oil
- Foaming soap container

Directions:

Mix in a bowl 5 parts water with one part of Castile soap, add in your essential oils. Add this mixture to foaming soap container. Shake well before using.

19. Vanilla & Lavender Detoxing Bath Salts
Ingredients:

- 10 drops of lavender essential oil
- 10 drops of vanilla essential oil
- 1.5 parts baking soda
- 2 parts sea salt
- 6 parts Epsom salts

Directions:

Place all the ingredients into a sealable container and shake well. Add about ½ a cup to your bath water. Soak and relax in your bath for at least 20 minutes.

20. Foaming Face Wash

Ingredients:

- 10 drops of Ylang Ylang essential oil
- 6 drops of patchouli essential oil
- ½ teaspoon almond oil or olive oil
- 2/3 cup distilled water
- 1/3 cup of castile soap
- 5 drops of lemongrass essential oil

Directions:

Pour the soap and oil into a foaming dispenser. Add in your essential oils and swirl to combine mixture. Fill the container with distilled water.

21. Bubble Bath

Ingredients:

- 10 drops of your favorite essential oil
- 2/3 cups of vegetable glycerin
- 1 cup of unscented Castile soap

Directions:

Mix ingredients in a sealable container. Add in 2 tablespoons to bath water while the water is running. Relax and soak for at least 20 minutes in your bubble bath and enjoy!

Chapter 3. Aromatherapy Essential Oil Blends

There are scientific reasons why aromatherapy works for humans. It is known that various scents will trigger many emotions and reactions in humans. When we are exposed to a scent, our nasal receptors sense it. They then send a signal to our brains and this helps trigger the centers of our brains which control memory, sensory perception, and thought processes. It also sends a signal to a gland in our brain that controls many of the chemicals that are coursing through our bodies, including serotonin which counteracts anxiety and endorphins which help reduce pain.

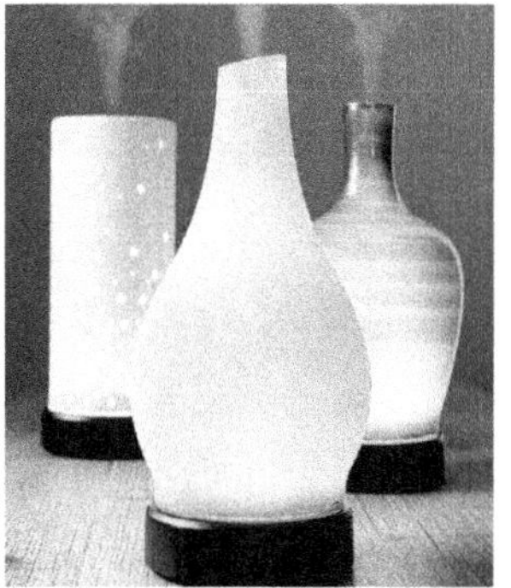

When we inhale essential oils, it is a good way for us to achieve emotional balance and to treat physical problems. You can either inhale essential oils directly or you can use a diffuser. With direct inhalation, you will receive quick relief. Just hold a bottle of essential oils under your nose and take a sniff while you breathe deeply.

Due to the volatile nature of essential oils using a diffuser makes is ideal for dispersing them into the air. When using a diffuser, it will gently heat up the oils to release their beneficial vapours into the air. What makes working with essential oils so wonderful is that you can personalize them to your special body chemistry. Research has shown that aromatherapy does have positive benefits such as relief from anxiety and depression, improving sleep, pain reduction and much more.

The aromatherapy oils are extracted from plants and distilled. These are highly concentrated oils that may be inhaled directly, or indirectly, and used in massage oils, lotions and bath salts. You can begin to tailor the oils to your personal needs once you begin to understand the characteristics of the oils.

Science is aware that there are subtle differences between these oils that can produce various reactions in the human body. Below are some of the benefits that essential oils offer.

Antidepressant

A widespread use in aromatherapy is in the treatment of depression. Instead of using pharmaceutical antidepressants try using chamomile, lavender, peppermint and jasmine. Treatment for severe depression should be done with a licensed practitioner.

Manage Energy Levels

All too often we use stimulants such as energy drinks and coffee, sugar and sports drinks to give us the boost we need when we are feeling low of energy. Instead, why not choose to use essential oils to increase your circulation and energy levels and help to stimulate your mind, without the dangerous side effects of chemicals. Uplifting essential oils include cinnamon, black pepper, clove, cardamom, jasmine, rosemary, and sage.

Healing

Many essential oils help with healing and recovery of injuries or surgery. These oils can help to stimulate oxygen and blood flow to wounds and some protect your body because of their anti-microbial properties. Some of the best essential oils for healing and recovery are lavender, rosehip, calendula, and buckthorn.

Headaches

Instead of grabbing a pill, why not try essential oils to ease your headache pain. Lying down in a cool, dark room while you inhale a few drops of peppermint, eucalyptus, rosemary or sandalwood essential oils are an excellent alternative to pills. You can mix the oils in a carrier oil such as coconut oil, almond oil, or avocado oil and use this to massage into your temples, scalp and neck.

Restore Sleep Rhythms

Sleep is vital for us to function properly, we must have proper sleep, during which time our bodies rebuild and restore cells and energy levels. Consider using aromatherapy if you have trouble falling asleep, it can help to promote rest. Try rose, lavender, sandalwood, chamomile, marjoram, neroli, Ylang Ylang essential oils.

Help to Boost Your Immune System

Many essential oils have anti-microbial, antibacterial, and antifungal effects that can help to protect you from infection and disease. When you use essential oils in your home you are not only avoiding toxic chemicals; you are also helping to cleanse the air and protect your body from harm. Try peppermint, lemon, oregano, frankincense, cinnamon, and eucalyptus essential oils to help give your immune system.

Pain Relief

Not everyone likes to take pills for pain and essential oils have been proven to help without the negative side effects of using chemicals. Essential oils used for pain relief include peppermint, lavender, chamomile, clary sage, rosemary, eucalyptus and juniper essential oils.

Stress Relief

The aromatic compounds in many essential oils can help to soothe your mind and are relaxants, and will help to eliminate anxiety. Some of the best essential oils for stress relief are lavender, lemon, and peppermint. There has been research that has shown lemon essential oil can improve mood and reduce outbursts of anger.

Pamper Yourself

Essential oils are great at absorbing into your skin and can cleanse, deodorize, tone and balance it. They are perfect to use during a massage, facial treatments, baths etc. They are wonderful to use on your skin which is the largest organ of your body. Your skin must endure the daily barrage of the surrounding environment it is in. UV damage, pollutants along with heat and cold all affect your skin. Essential oils can be used to help restore balance. Lavender essential oil is one of the best essential oils to use.

The following blends are meant to be used in a cold-air diffuser. These diffusers usually require you to add a small amount of water to the oils. Follow the directions of the manufacturer of your diffuser. Tailor these mixtures to suit your personal tastes and needs.

22. Fresh and Clean Essential Oil Diffuser Recipe
Ingredients:

- 2 drops lemon essential oil
- 3 drops of lavender essential oil
- 2 drops of rosemary essential oil

Directions:

Add ingredients to your diffuser per the manufacturer's instructions of your diffuser.

23. Seasonal Allergies Essential Oil Diffuser Recipe

Ingredients:

- 3 drops of lemon essential oil
- 3 drops of lavender essential oil
- 2 drops of peppermint essential oil

Directions:

Add ingredients to your diffuser per the manufacturer's instructions of your diffuser.

24. Flower Garden Essential Oil Diffuser Recipe
Ingredients:

- 2 drops of lavender essential oil
- 2 drops of geranium essential oil
- 2 drops of roman chamomile essential oil

Directions:

Add ingredients to your diffuser per the manufacturer's instructions of your diffuser.

25. Morning Boost Essential Oil Diffuser Recipe

Ingredients:

- 2 drops of cinnamon essential oil
- 2 drops of frankincense essential oil
- 2 drops of wild orange essential oil

Directions:

Add ingredients to your diffuser per the manufacturer's instructions of your diffuser.

26. Cold and Flu Season Essential Oil Diffuser Recipe

Ingredients:

- 1 drop of wild orange essential oil
- 1 drop of cinnamon bark essential oil
- 1 drop clove essential oil
- 1 drop eucalyptus essential oil
- 1 drop rosemary essential oil

Directions:

Add ingredients to your diffuser per the manufacturer's instructions of your diffuser.

27. Focus and Alertness Essential Oil Diffuser Recipe

Ingredients:

- 2 drops of peppermint essential oil
- 2 drops of wild orange essential oil
- 2 drops of lemon essential oil

Directions:

Add ingredients to your diffuser per the manufacturer's instructions of your diffuser.

28. *Odor Eliminator Essential Oil Diffuser Recipe*

Ingredients:

- 1 drop of lime essential oil
- 1 drop of cilantro essential oil
- 1 drop of melaleuca essential oil
- 2 drops of lemon essential oil

Directions:

Add ingredients to your diffuser per the manufacturer's instructions of your diffuser.

Chapter 4. DIY Budget Friendly Cleaning Products

You can easily make your own cleaning products for your kitchen and save money while you improve your health. Using simple ingredients such as essential oils, vinegar, water and baking soda are all healthy and cheap ingredients.

29. Vinyl & Linoleum
Ingredients:

- 1 gallon of warm water
- 3 drops of lemon essential oil
- 1 cup of vinegar

Directions:

Mix all of the ingredients in a bucket and use this to clean your vinyl and linoleum floors with.

30. Dusting Spray

Ingredients:

- ¼ cup of olive oil
- 2 tablespoons of lemon juice
- 5 drops of lemon essential oil

Directions:

Add all the ingredients into a spray bottle and shake well before using. Spray mix onto a cloth and wipe down surface.

31. Wood Polish

Ingredients:

- 1 tablespoon of olive oil
- ¾ cup of water
- 2 tablespoons of white vinegar
- 1 tablespoon of liquid glycerin
- 40 drops of lemon or orange essential oil
- ¼ teaspoon of Xanthan gum
- ½ teaspoon Emulsifying wax

Directions:

Put the essential oils, water, glycerine and vinegar into blender and blend these ingredients on high speed. Add in the emulsifying wax and Xanthan gum while motor is running. Process mixture for about 15 seconds to make it slightly thick. Pour in one spritz bottle and use once a week. This can be kept for almost three months.

32. Simple Dusting Spray

Ingredients:

- ¾ cup of olive oil
- ¼ cup of distilled vinegar
- 40 drops of lemon, clove or orange essential oil

Directions:

Add all the ingredients into a spray bottle and spray mix onto dry cloth and apply to furniture.

Chapter 5. Teeth Cleaners & More!

33. Squeezable Toothpaste for Clean Teeth

Ingredients:

- 20 drops of peppermint essential oil
- 5 drops of fennel essential oil
- 1 teaspoon miswak powder or whole ground stevia powder
- ½ teaspoon baking soda
- 1 teaspoon sea salt
- 6 tablespoons of bentonite clay
- 4 tablespoons of coconut oil

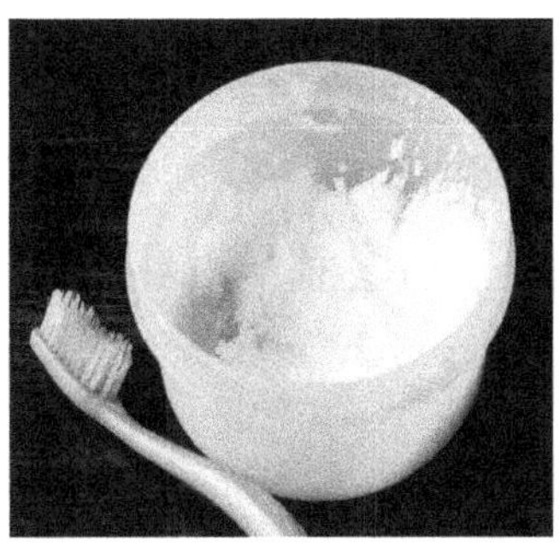

Directions:

To make your toothpaste thick, keep adding distilled water, tsp by tsp. Blend all your ingredients in a mixing bowl. Once you have reached the consistency you desire. Transfer the toothpaste into squeezable tubes.

34. Teeth Whitening Scrub

Ingredients:

- 1 drop of lemon essential oil
- 2 drops of peppermint essential oil
- ½ teaspoon of honey
- ½ teaspoon of bentonite clay
- ½ teaspoon of baking soda

Directions:

In a small dish combine your ingredients, blend them well. Apply the paste onto your teeth and leave on for 10 minutes. Rinse your mouth with tepid water.

35. Detox Bath Recipe

Ingredients:

- 6 drops of lavender essential oil
- 5 drops of cedarwood essential oil
- 3 drops of ginger essential oil
- 1 tablespoon of coconut oil
- ¼ cup baking soda
- Handful of Epsom salts

Directions:

Mix ingredients in a bowl and then add them to a hot bath. Have a nice long 30-minute soak to detox your entire system.

36. Detox Hair Mask

Ingredients:

- 4 drops of tea tree essential oil
- 5 drops of eucalyptus essential oil
- 7 drops of thyme essential oil
- 1 teaspoon of raw apple cider vinegar
- 1 tablespoon of marshmallow root powder
- ¾ cup bentonite clay

Directions:

Mix the ingredients in a bowl, adding water to help form a paste. Apply a thick coat of the paste over your hair and scalp. Allow it to penetrate for about 15-minutes. Rinse it off with tepid water. Once it is rinsed out, do a final rinse using cold water, then wrap your hair in a nice soft towel.

37. Powerful Essential Oil Blend for Toenail Fungus
Ingredients:

- 3 drops each of thyme, oregano, and clove essential oils
- Amber glass dropper bottle

Directions:

Mix the blend in the amber glass dropper bottle. Apply one drop of this powerful blend on the infected toenail. Allow the antifungal blend to sink deeper into toenail, sit still for at least ten minutes during this process.

38. Foot Soak

Ingredients:

- 10 drops of winter savory essential oil
- 5 teaspoons of sea salt
- Tub or basin to soak feet in

Directions:

Fill the basin with hot water, add in your ingredients and stir well. Soak your feet for about 20 minutes.

39. Healing Blend for Acne Scars

Ingredients:

- 10 drops of Helichrysum essential oil
- 10 drops of frankincense essential oil
- 10 drops of lavender essential oil
- 1 ounce of rosehip essential oil

Directions:

Add your essential oils into an amber glass dropper bottle. Massage a few drops of this blend to area of skin that has acne scars, it will help to fade the scars.

40. Pumpkin Spice Scrub Cubes
Ingredients:

- ¼ cup of coconut oil
- ½ cup of grated unscented soap
- 1 teaspoon of pumpkin spice
- 5 drops of cinnamon essential oil
- 5 drops of sweet orange essential oil
- 3 drops of cedarwood essential oil

Directions:

In a double boiler, melt the shredded soap base and ¼ cup of coconut oil. Remove from heat after melted, add in the remaining ingredients and stir until well blended. Quickly pour mixture into silicone molds and allow to freeze for an hour or two.

41. Exfoliating Lip Scrub
Ingredients:

- 3 drops of cinnamon essential oil
- 2 tablespoons of raw honey
- 3 tablespoons of brown sugar

Directions:

Mix your ingredients in a small bowl. Scrub onto your lips. Leave it on for 5 minutes, and then rinse off with warm water.

42. Tea Tree Dandruff Shampoo

Ingredients:

- 15 drops of tea tree essential oil
- 1 teaspoon of fractionated coconut oil
- 2 tablespoons of Aloe Vera juice
- 1/3 cup of liquid Castile soap
- Soap dispenser bottle

Directions:

Add your ingredients into your soap dispenser, top it off with distilled water. Shake well to combine ingredients. Lather up your scalp and hair with this shampoo to get rid of the dandruff.

43. Facial Mist for Radiant Skin

Ingredients:

- 1 tablespoon of Aloe Vera juice
- 15 drops of rose essential oil
- ¾ cup of rose water
- 8-ounce spray bottle

Directions:

Add your ingredients to your spray bottle and shake well. Spritz this blend onto your face to refresh your facial skin.

44. Foaming Citrus Body Wash
Ingredients:

- Distilled water
- 7 drops of bergamot essential oil
- 10 drops of grapefruit essential oil
- 2 tablespoon of vegetable glycerine
- 1 tablespoon of fractionated coconut oil
- 2 tablespoons of jojoba oil
- ½ cup of liquid Castile soap

Directions:

Add all your ingredients into a soap dispenser, and top off with distilled water. Shake well before each use.

45. Skin Clearing Facial Mask
Ingredients:

- 3 drops of tea tree essential oil
- 1 teaspoon of coconut oil
- 2 teaspoons of oat flour

Directions:

Mix your ingredients in a small bowl. Once your mixture is creamy in texture, apply it to your face. Leave it on for 5 minutes. Rinse mask off, using warm water and pat dry with a face towel.

Conclusion

I hope that you and your loved ones will enjoy trying and using my collection of essential oil cleaners for keeping both your bodies and home environment safe and clean. I am sure you are going to be so glad that you decided to make this important positive step in life, by turning away from those harmful chemical-filled cleaning products on the market and replacing them with natural home cleaning products that are good for your health and the environments! That my friend is what I call a win-win situation!

I would like to thank you once again for downloading my book, and showing support of my work. I greatly appreciate your support, and would really love to read a review of my book by you on Amazon!

FREE Bonus Reminder

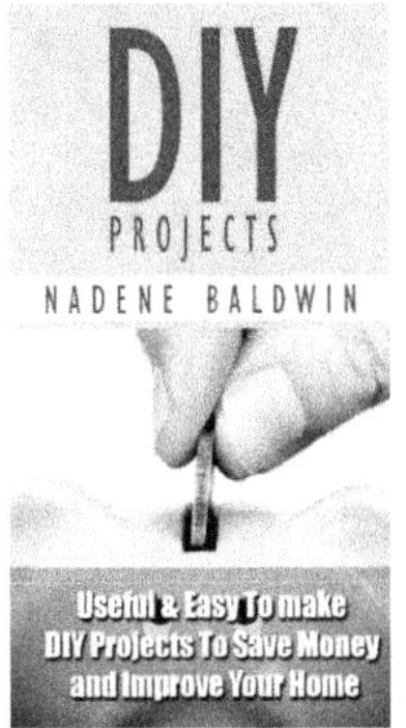

If you have not grabbed it yet, please go ahead and download your special bonus report *"DIY Projects. 13 Useful & Easy To Make DIY Projects To Save Money & Improve Your Home!"*
Simply Click the Button Below

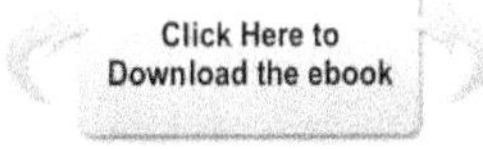

OR **Go to This Page**
http://diyhomecraft.com/free

BONUS #2: More Free & Discounted Books or Products

Do you want to receive more Free/Discounted Books or Products?
We have a mailing list where we send out our new Books or Products when they go free or with a discount on Amazon. Click on the link below to sign up for Free & Discount Book & Product Promotions.
=> Sign Up for Free & Discount Book & Product Promotions <=

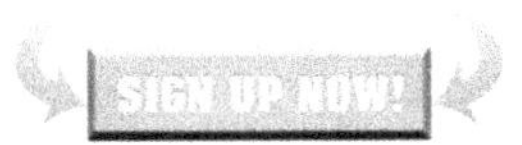

OR Go to this URL
http://bit.ly/1WBb1Ek